Hattie's Journey

A Child's Second Chance at Life After a Kidney Transplant

By
Dr. Felicia Williams-McGowan

Copyright © 2015 Opportune Independent Publishing Company

All rights reserved. No part of this publication may be reproduced, distributed, or transmitted in any form or by any means, including photocopying, recording, or other electronic or mechanical methods, without the prior written permission of the publisher, except in the case of brief quotations embodied in critical reviews and certain other noncommercial uses permitted by copyright law.

ISBN 10: 0996569448

ISBN 13: 978-0-9965694-4-6

Published by Opportune Independent Publishing Co.

Illustration by Keira LaRaque

Printed in the United States of America

For permission requests, write to the publisher, addressed "Attention: Permissions Coordinator," at the address below.

info@opportunepublishing.com

www.opportunepublishing.com

Disclaimer

Although the author and publisher have made every effort to ensure that the information in this book was correct at press time, the author and publisher do not assume and hereby disclaim any liability to any party for any loss, damage, or disruption caused by errors or omissions, whether such errors or omissions result from negligence, accident, or any other cause.

Dedication

First, I would like to give thanks to the Almighty. He has truly been my strength through this journey. To my mother, Hattie Lee Osborne (Armetta) Williams, without you sacrificing your life for mine I would not have this story to tell. You have supported me through all of my endeavors, which has given me the strength to accomplish my goals and dreams. To my father for always having high expectations of me. You did not give me the opportunity to quit and you always believed that I would exceed in anything I wanted to achieve. I love you both! To my husband, thank you for your support. To all of my family and friends for your encouragement through all the battles I had to fight. The end result was worth it all!

The News

It was the second day of school, the sun was shining and the birds were singing in the trees. As the clock struck eight o'clock, Hattie didn't spring up as she normally does. She told her mom that she didn't feel well at all. She was very tired and couldn't move without being in pain.

So, to the doctor's office they went.

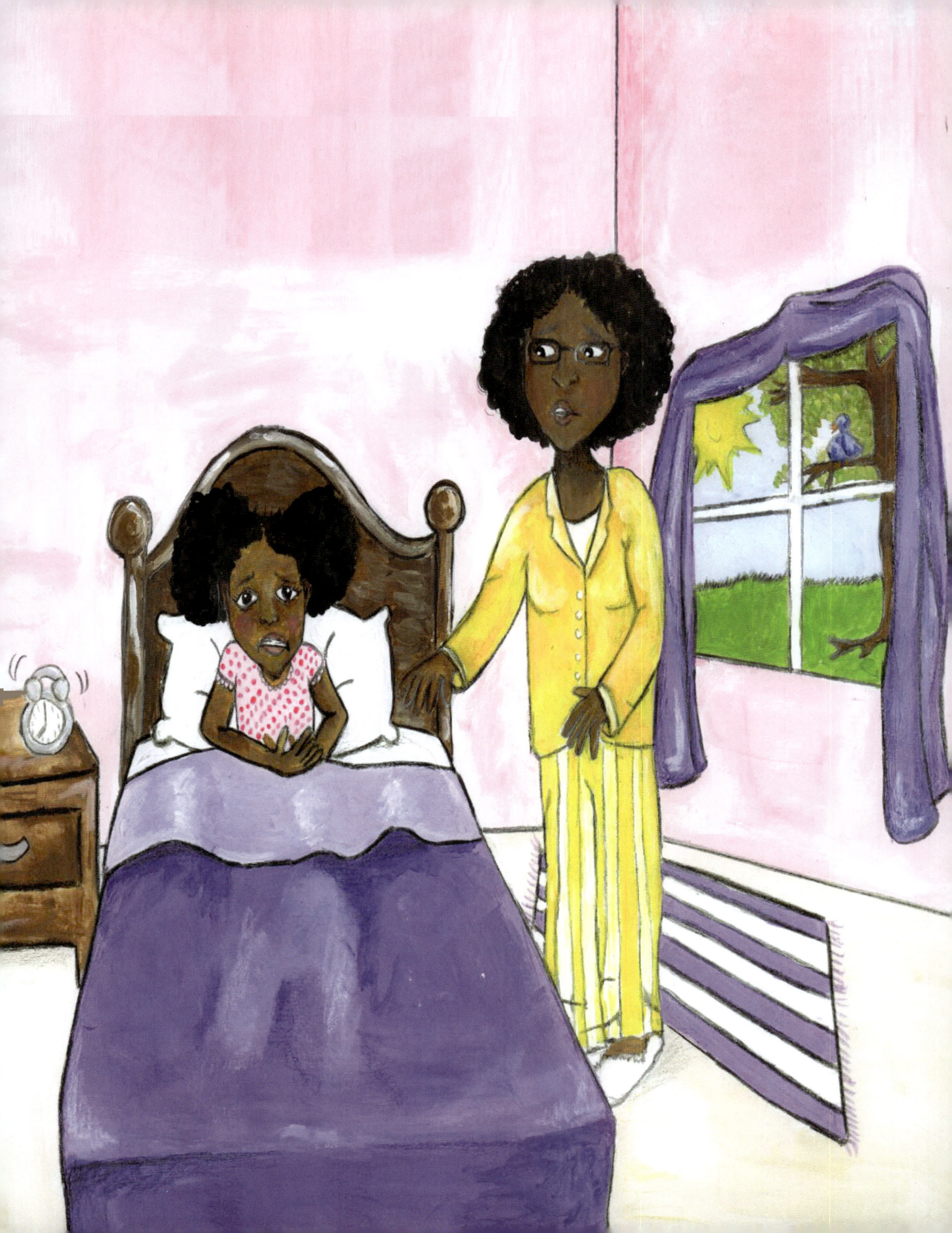

She saw Dr. Middle, who sent her to see Dr. Left. Then she saw Dr. Right. After each doctor ran tests and asked questions, they still couldn't find out what was wrong with Hattie. After many attempts, they sent her home in hopes that rest would help her feel better.

On Friday, Hattie was on her way to cheer at a football game. She had her uniform on and pom poms at her side. While getting out of the car she felt the most intense pain she'd ever felt in her life. She grabbed her stomach with both arms and could barely stand up straight.

Her mom could see the agony she was in and immediately drove her to the nearest hospital. While in the waiting room, Hattie cried out "I feel really bad mom."

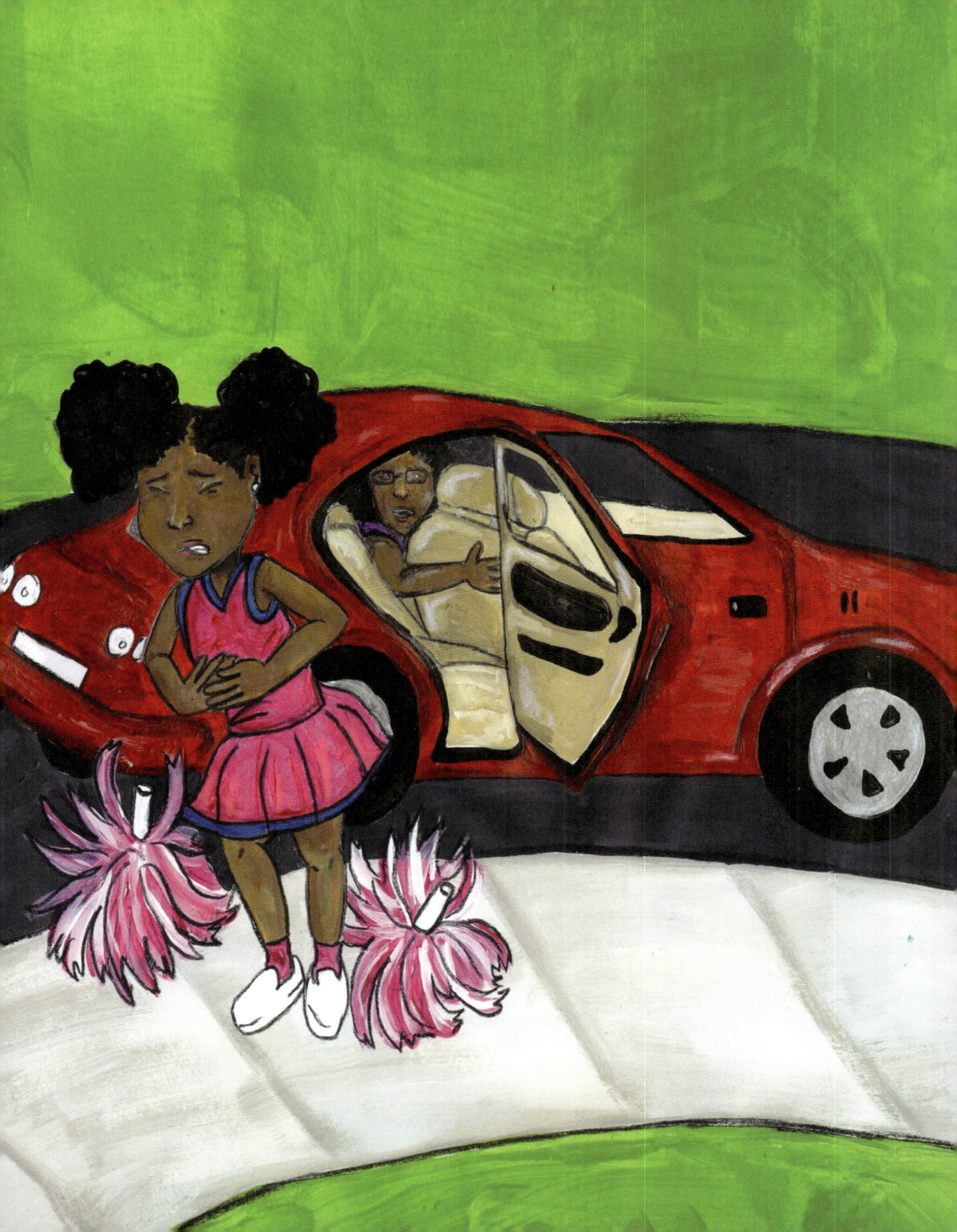

The doctors at the local hospital sent Hattie to a kidney specialist at Destunee Medical. Dr. Biggs ordered many tests and kept her overnight to figure out exactly what was wrong with her.

The next morning, Dr. Biggs explained that all the pain that Hattie was in was because she had Kidney failure.

"What does that mean?" The family asked.

Dr. Biggs told the family that having kidney disease means that your body cannot get rid of all the toxins and bad stuff when going to the restroom. "This is a very serious condition," the doctor explained. Kidney failure increases the risk of other problems with your body if not given the proper care.

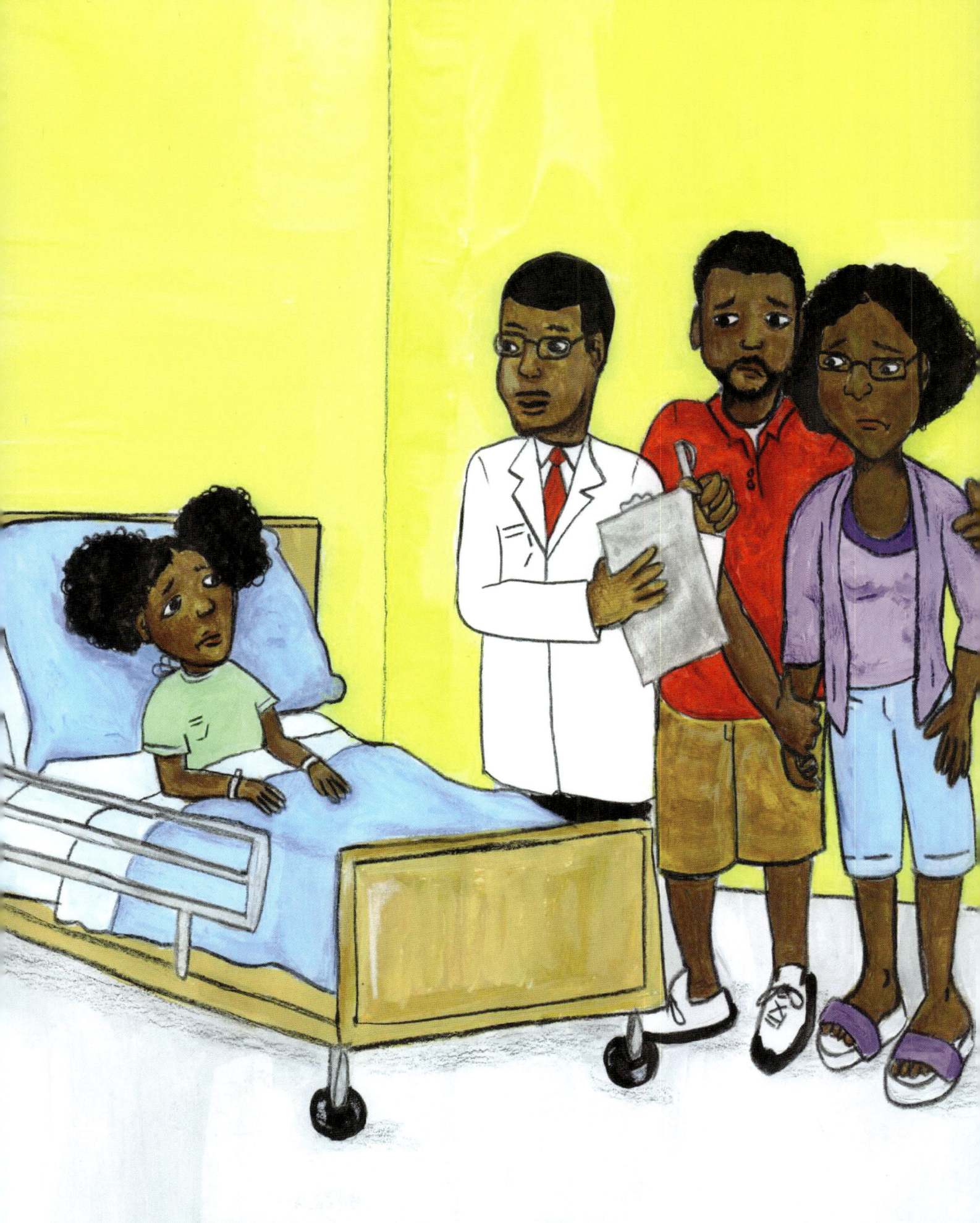

Hattie and her family were so confused. No one had ever heard of this Kidney disease, nor did they know how Hattie had gotten it. Dr. Biggs told the family that Hattie's kidneys had completely failed and she would have to start treatment for this immediately.

"What should we do?" asked her father.

Dr. Biggs explained to the family that Hattie will need to go on peritioneal dialysis.

Dialysis

The next day Hattie woke up in the hospital room with tears rolling down her eyes looking out the window. The sun was beaming on her toffee skin and all she could think about was, "What will my life be like? Why do I have to go through this? Will the other kids laugh at me?"

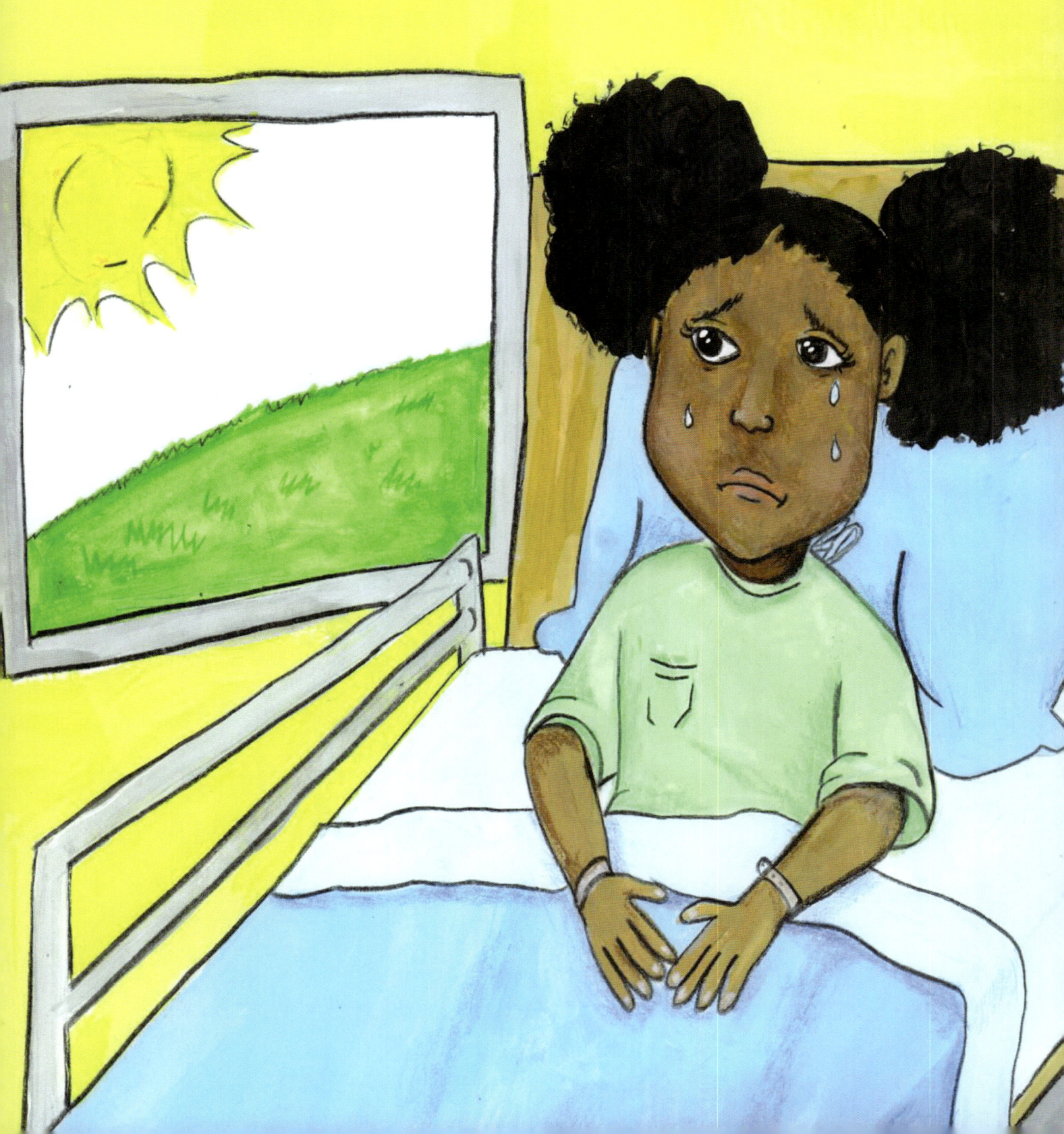

The first step was to have surgery so Hattie could begin her dialysis treatment. As the nurses came into the room to prepare her for the operation, Nurse Little smiled and said, "Everything would be fine, I promise."

After the surgery, Dr. Biggs came to Hattie's room and began to train everyone on how to take care of Hattie going forward. When dialysis treatments begin Hattie will wear bags that are connected to her stomach. The bags will have to be switched out 5 times a day. Next, she would have to take medicine every single day to keep her well. But the worst part was yet to come.

Dr. Biggs then said the words no kid wants to hear, "You can no longer eat whatever you want." Hattie's diet would need to be free of salt and limited fluid intake. All she heard was "No more French fries and milkshakes."

The information was concerning to Hattie and her

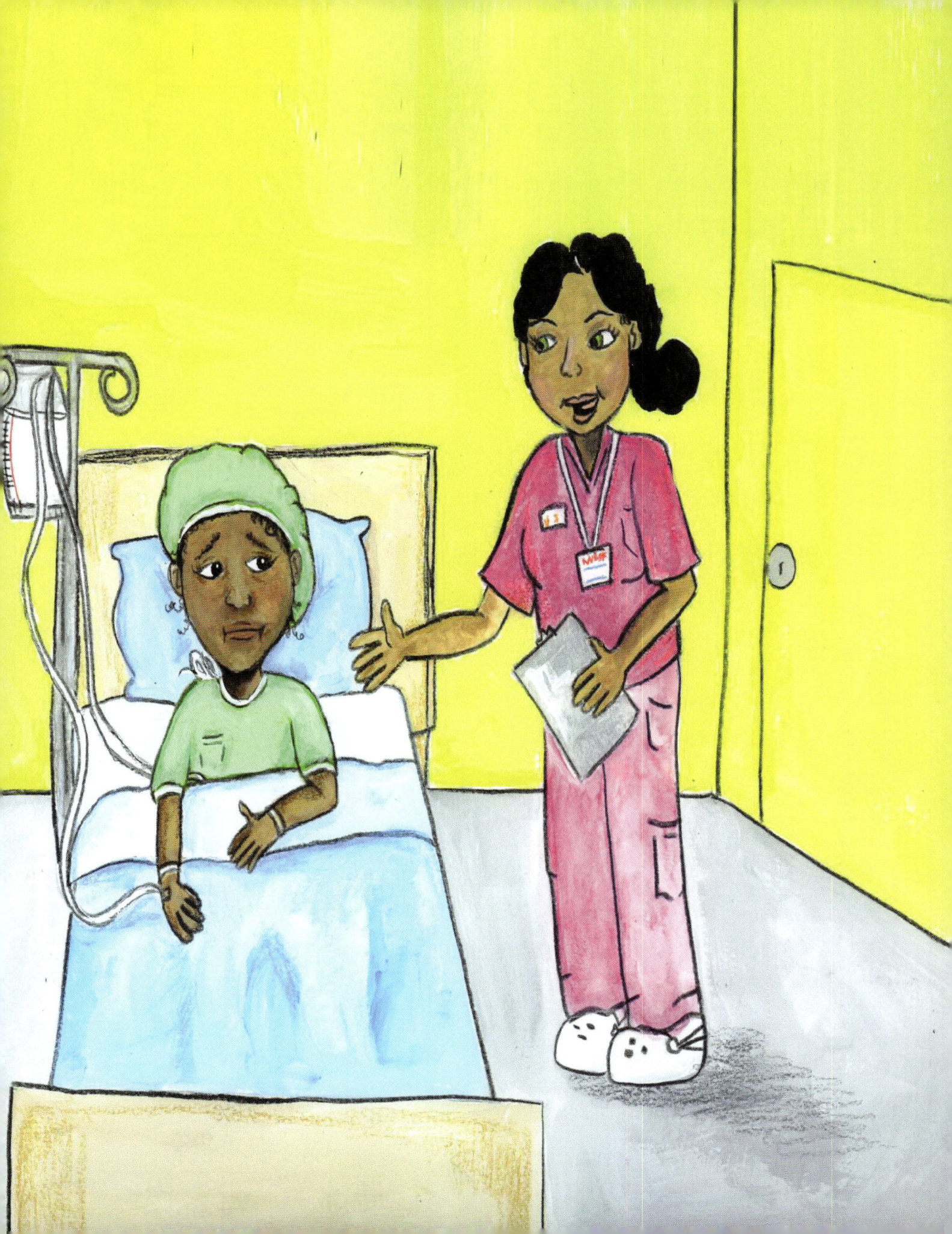

family. Hattie asked the doctor, "Can I go to school" and will the other kids know I have a bag on me?" School was Hattie's favorite place to be, she was a cheerleader and very popular in school.

Dr. Biggs explained to Hattie that she could not cheer while on dialysis. Hattie felt a lump in her throat and she could not believe what her ears were hearing. Hattie looked down at the tube that had been placed in her stomach. "This is going to ruin my life," Hattie thought.

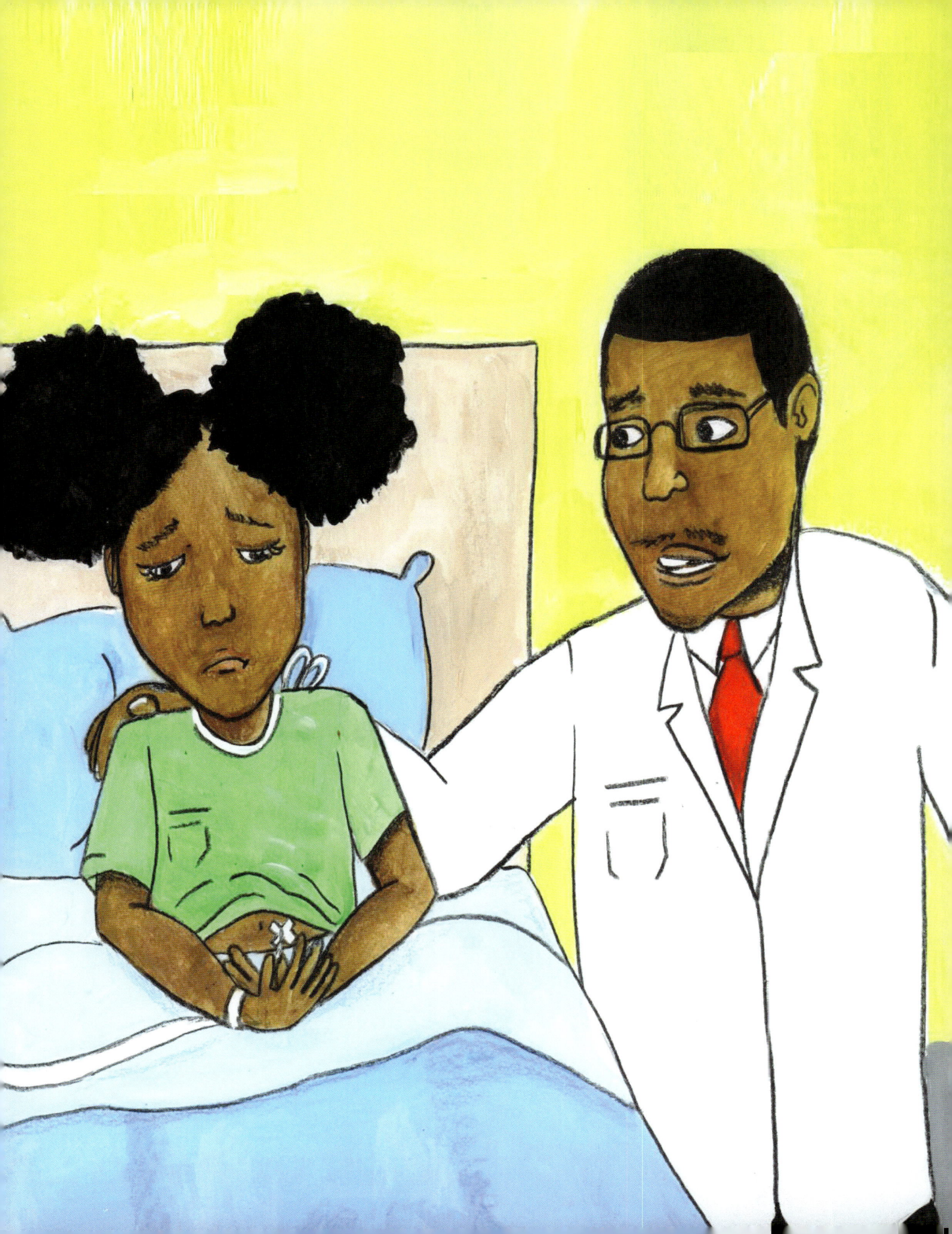

Hattie was very weak and had to be on homebound for the first part of the semester.

Hattie was very strong willed and at twelve she was not going to give up her life for this disease. After thinking about the changes that were happening in her life, Hattie was ready to take on the world and take care of herself. All she wanted was to feel better and be with her family and friends. While on dialysis Hattie was able to do just that.

Even though Hattie was disappointed that she could not cheer anymore it was agreed upon that she could be a manager for the basketball team. Hattie could go home to eat her special diet and do dialysis during her scheduled lunchtime at school. Hattie did not imagine her life being this way, but nothing was going to stop her from enjoying her life, not even dialysis.

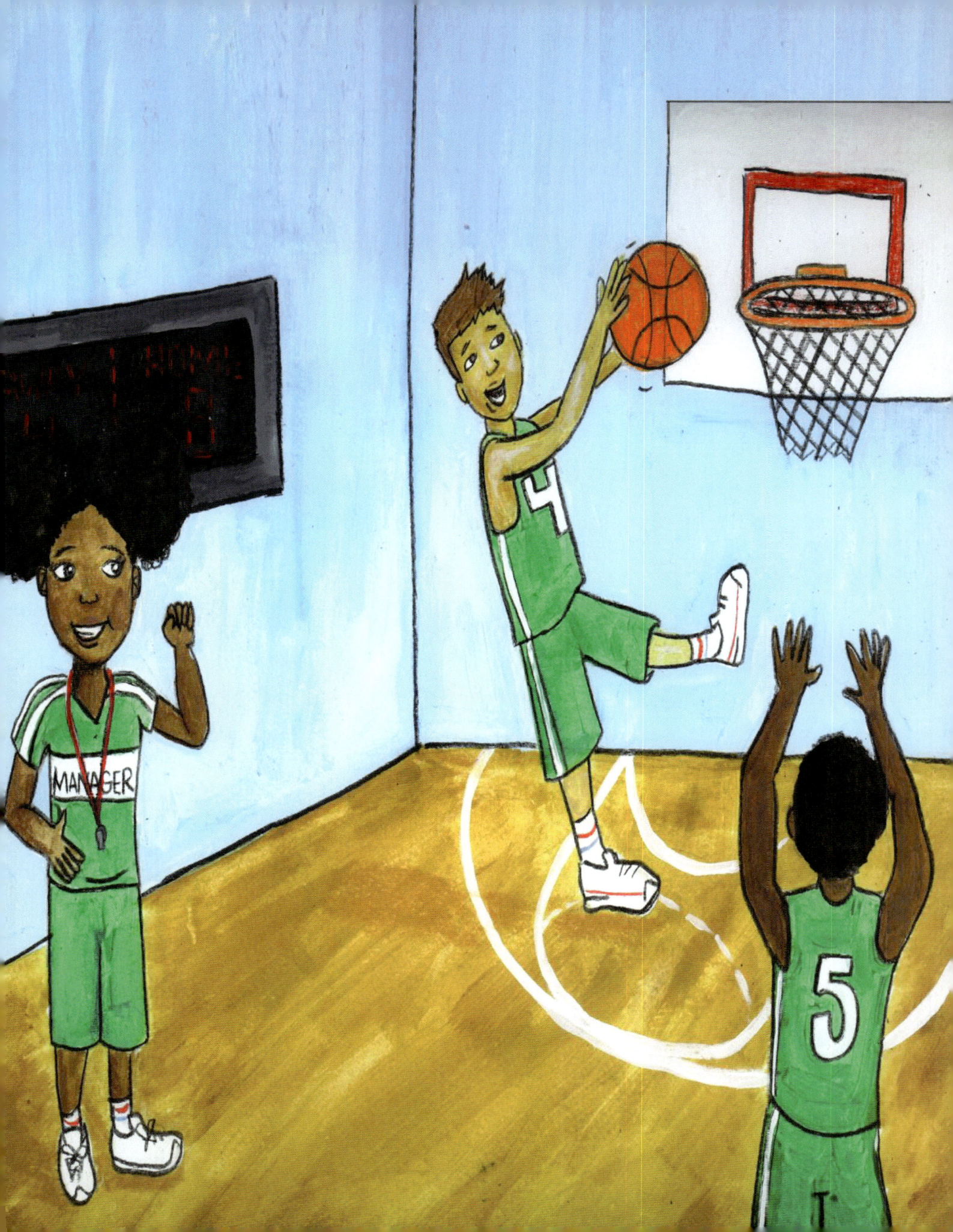

Transplant

Even though dialysis has worked to help clean the toxins, Hattie needed a new kidney to have a healthier lifestyle.

"How can I have a healthier lifestyle?" asked Hattie.
Dr. Briggs explained to Hattie that she would need a kidney transplant. This is when you receive a kidney from someone else.

Hattie's family wasn't sure about this transplant, because of all the expenses and how it could affect their family. Hattie's mom was willing to do anything for her baby.

Hattie's mom and dad were both tested to see if they matched. As a result of Hattie's dad not having excellent health, her mom was the best candidate for the surgery.

While other children her age were attending summer

camps, visiting family members and hanging out with friends. Hattie and her mother were attending doctors' appointments and having blood tests completed to make sure the transplant would be a success.

The day of the transplant surgery had finally come. It was hot and humid with a downpour of rain. But Hattie still had a reason to smile. She left home that morning grinning from ear to ear, because she knew that her life was getting ready to be changed for the better.

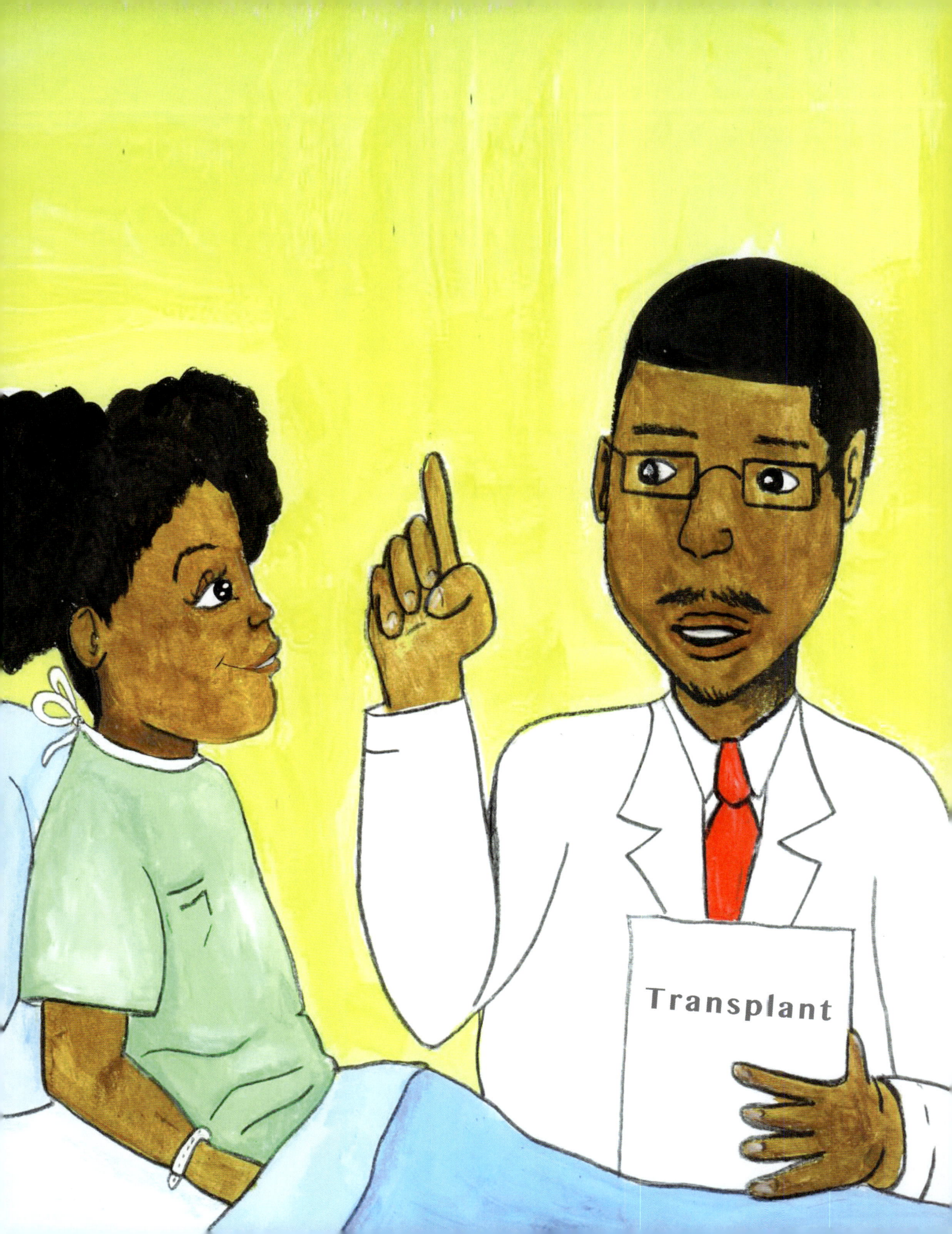

The surgery was successful!!

Hattie did so well that she was visiting her mothers' hospital room. Hattie told her parents, "I feel like a new person", mama I love you!" Thank you for giving me a second chance at life."

Soon, things started to get back to normal and life was even better than before.

Hattie was attending school. She had planned to tryout for cheerleading and hangout with her friends.

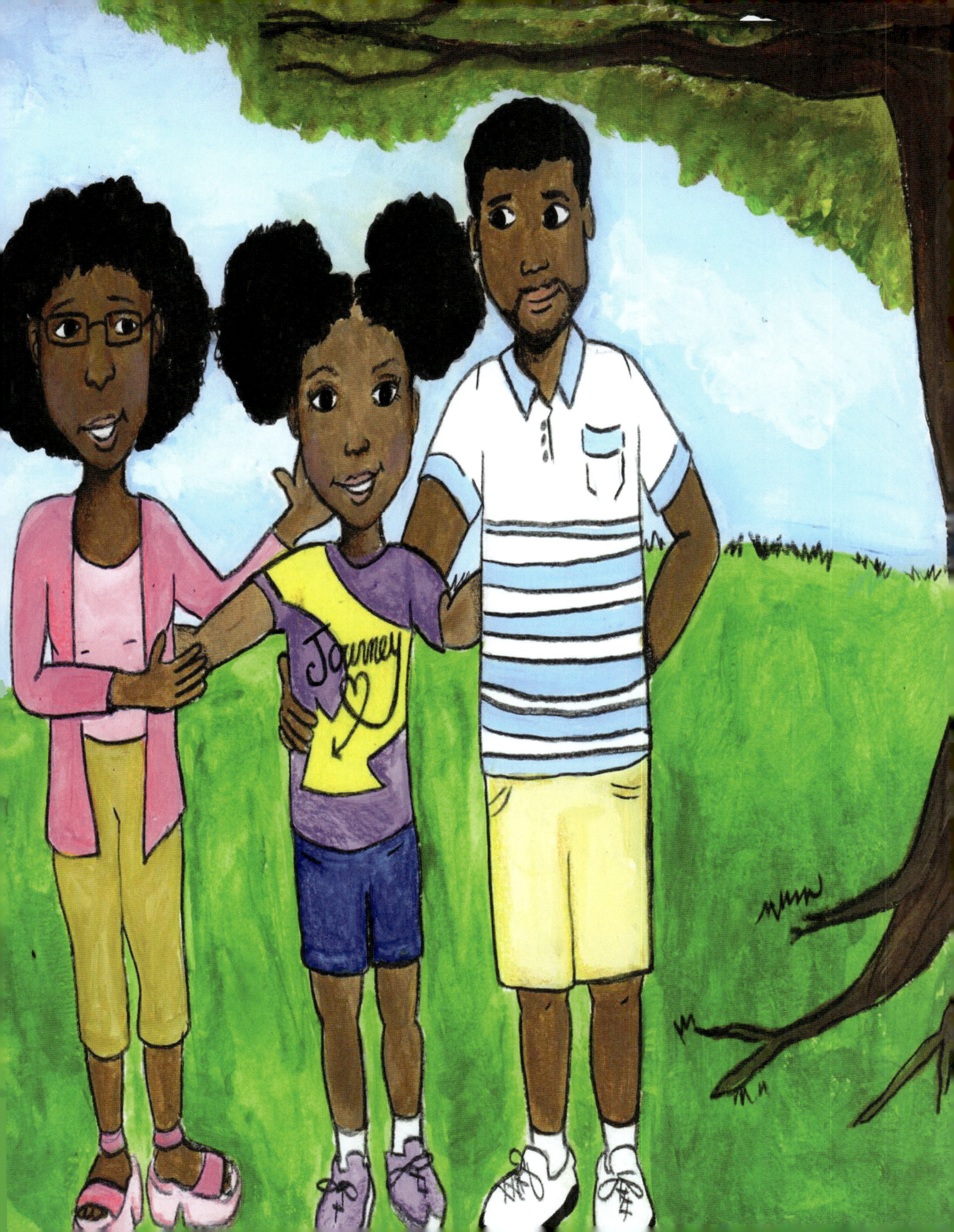

When Hattie's freshman year began at school she looked like a new person with a new attitude. Her face had a glow to it, and she was standing up straight and proud. When Hattie arrived to school in her new car that her father had given her, it was like she had not missed a thing. As she walked to her homeroom class a breeze blew across her face. She looked up in the sky as a reverence of being thankful for everything that she had gone through.

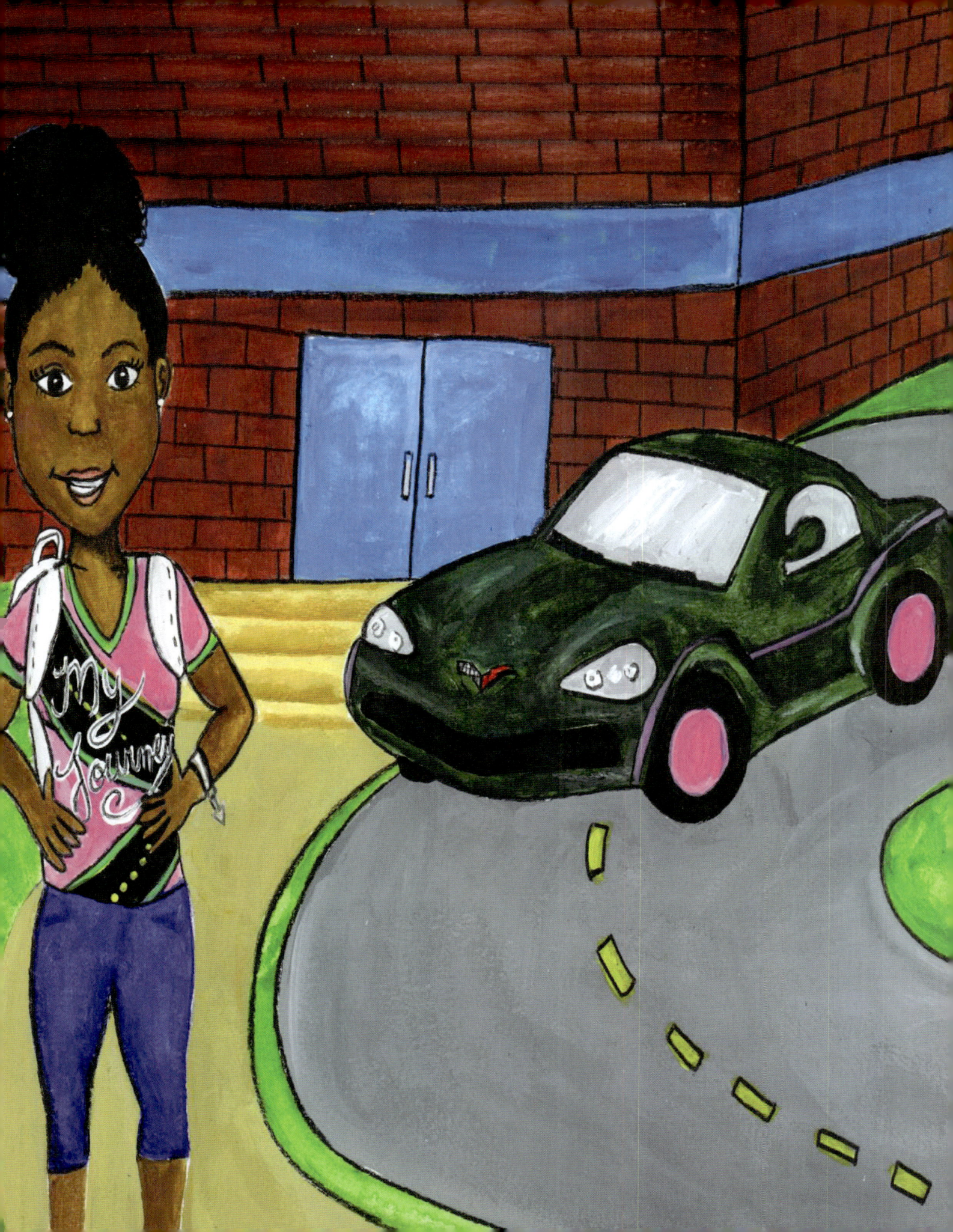

Although she had a new kidney and was no longer on dialysis, she still had to take care of one thing. Hattie needed to make sure she took her medicine as scheduled in order to keep her kidney healthy and stay well.

Being diagnosed with kidney failure was not just a disease for Hattie, but a lifestyle change. Hattie did not know what the future would bring, but she understood and knew that her life could only get better from here.

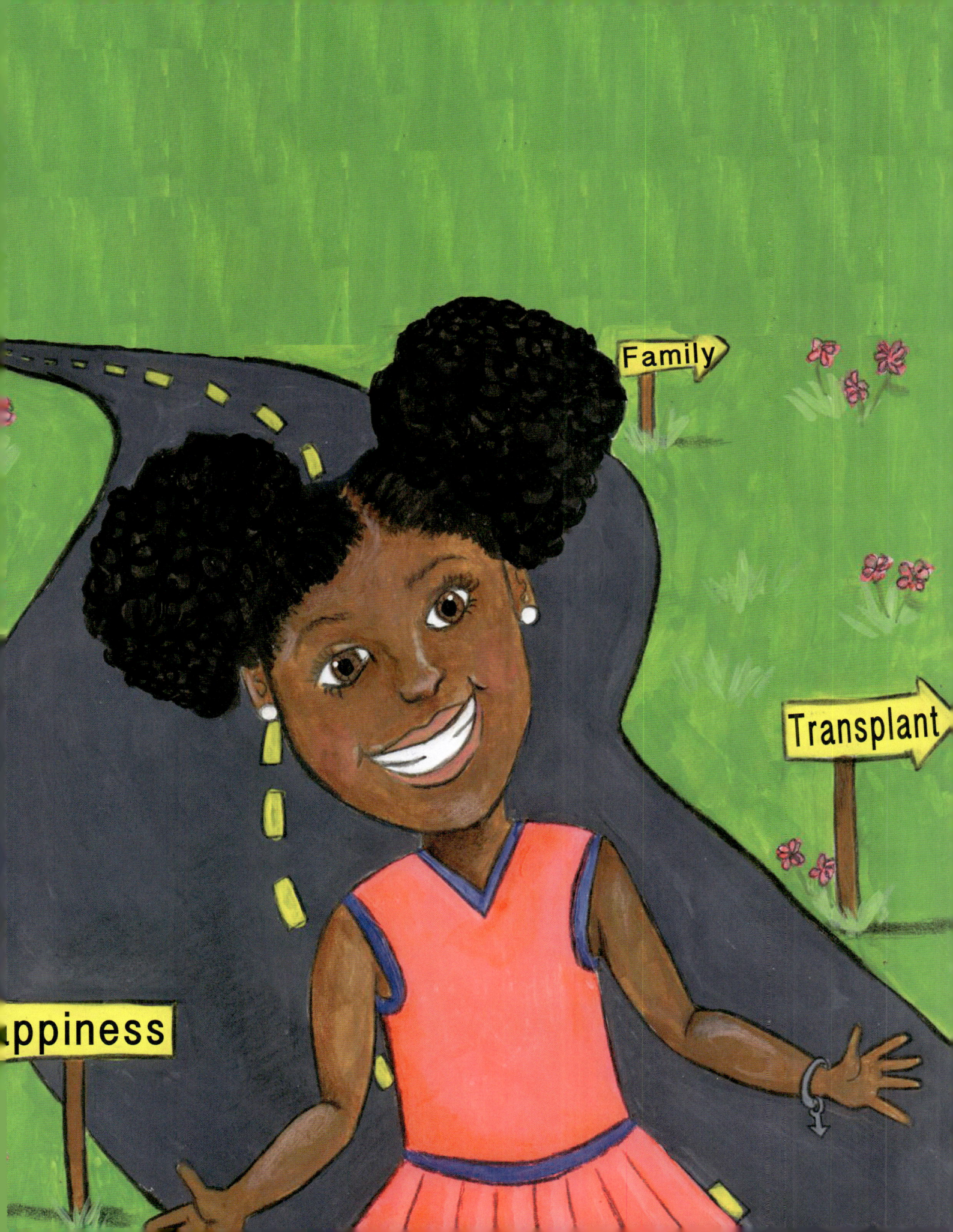

The story that has included the topic of **kidney transplantation** and **dialysis** which may be new to some readers. This researched information will give you a better understanding of what **kidney failure**, transplant and dialysis means.

Kidney failure described as end-stage **kidney disease** or ESRD when treated with a **kidney transplant** or blood-filtering treatments called dialysis—means the kidneys no longer work well enough to do their job. In most cases, **kidney failure** in children is treated with a **kidney transplant**. Though some children receive a **kidney transplant** before their kidneys fail completely, many children begin with dialysis to stay healthy until they can have a transplant.

Dialysis is the process of filtering wastes and extra fluid from the body by means other than the kidneys. Sometimes, a **transplanted kidney** may stop working, and the child may need to return to dialysis. Transplantation may be delayed if a matching kidney is not available or if the child has an infectious disease or an active **kidney disease** that has progressed rapidly.

Peritoneal dialysis uses the lining of the abdominal cavity—the space in the body that holds organs such as the stomach, intestines, and liver—to filter the blood. The lining is called the peritoneum. A kind of salty water called dialysis solution is emptied from a plastic bag through a catheter—a thin, flexible tube—into the abdominal cavity. While it is inside, the **dialysis** solution soaks up wastes and extra fluid from the body. After a few hours, the used **dialysis** solution is drained into another bag, removing the wastes and extra fluid from the body. The abdomen is filled with fluid all day and all night, so the filtering process never stops. The process of draining and refilling, called an exchange, takes about 30 minutes.

Kidney transplantation is surgery to place a healthy kidney from someone who has just died or a living donor, usually a family member, into a person's body to take over the job of the failing kidney. Once kidneys fail because of chronic **kidney disease** (CKD), function cannot be restored, so transplantation is the closest thing to a cure. Children with a transplant will need to take medications every day to prevent their body from rejecting the new kidney and get regular checkups to make sure the new kidney is accepted and functioning properly.

National Institute of Diabetes and Digestive and Kidney Disease (March 12, 2014). *Treatment Of Methods of Kidney Transplants in Children.* http://www.niddk.nih.gov/health-information/health-topics/kidney-disease/treatment-methods-for-kidney-failure-in-children/Pages/facts.aspx#2

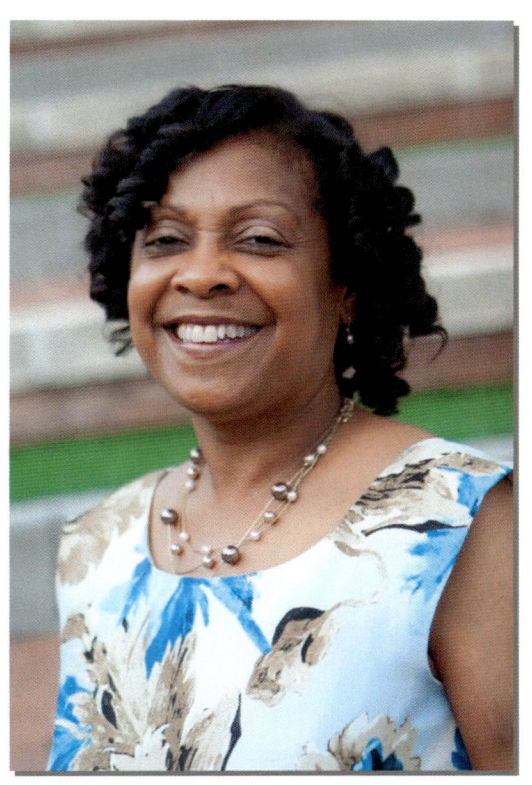

Dr. Felicia Arnetta Williams McGowan has been a school counselor for over 10 years in South Carolina. Dr. Williams McGowan was diagnosed with Kidney disease over 32 years ago which did not stop her from achieving educationally She has a Master in Mental Health Counseling with a certification in school counseling. She also has doctorate in educational leadership.

Hattie's Journey is a story of a little girl who loved school and all things fun. Experiencing a roadblock in her journey caused Hattie to reroute her path. Was Hattie able to overcome these obstacles in her life? *Hattie's Journey* is a children's book that can be used to familiarize readers of the different ups and downs families could face when a child has been diagnosed with kidney failure.

Williams McGowan authored her book *Hattie's Journey* because of her passion to bring awareness about kidney disease/transplantation and how it affects children. Her experiences with kidney disease led her to have a different life. Even with this way of life Dr. McGowan, her family, and friends created an environment to make sure her childhood was as normal as possible. Dr. Felicia Williams-McGowan quotes "No matter how short no matter how long keep traveling through your journey."

Coloring Book

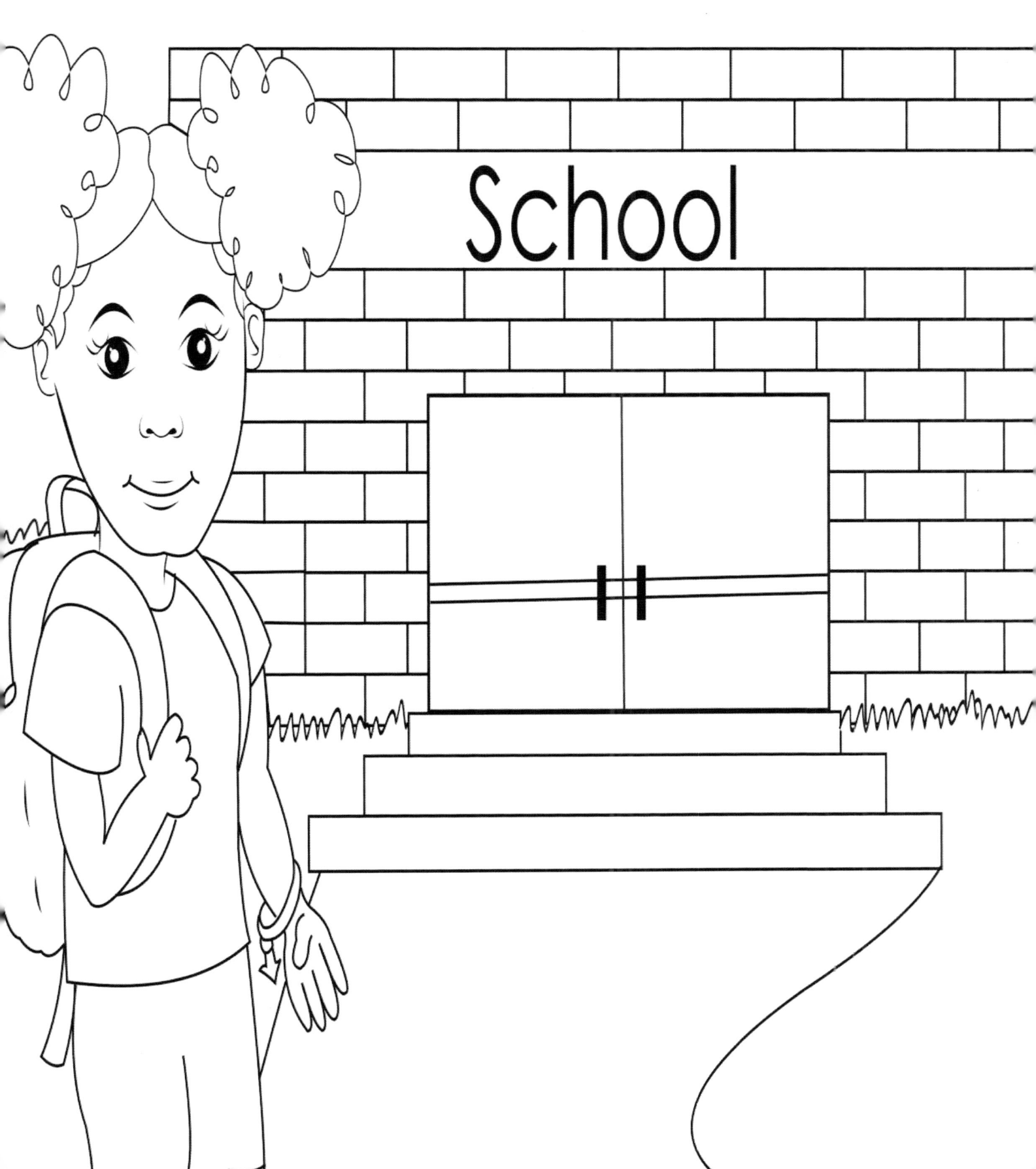

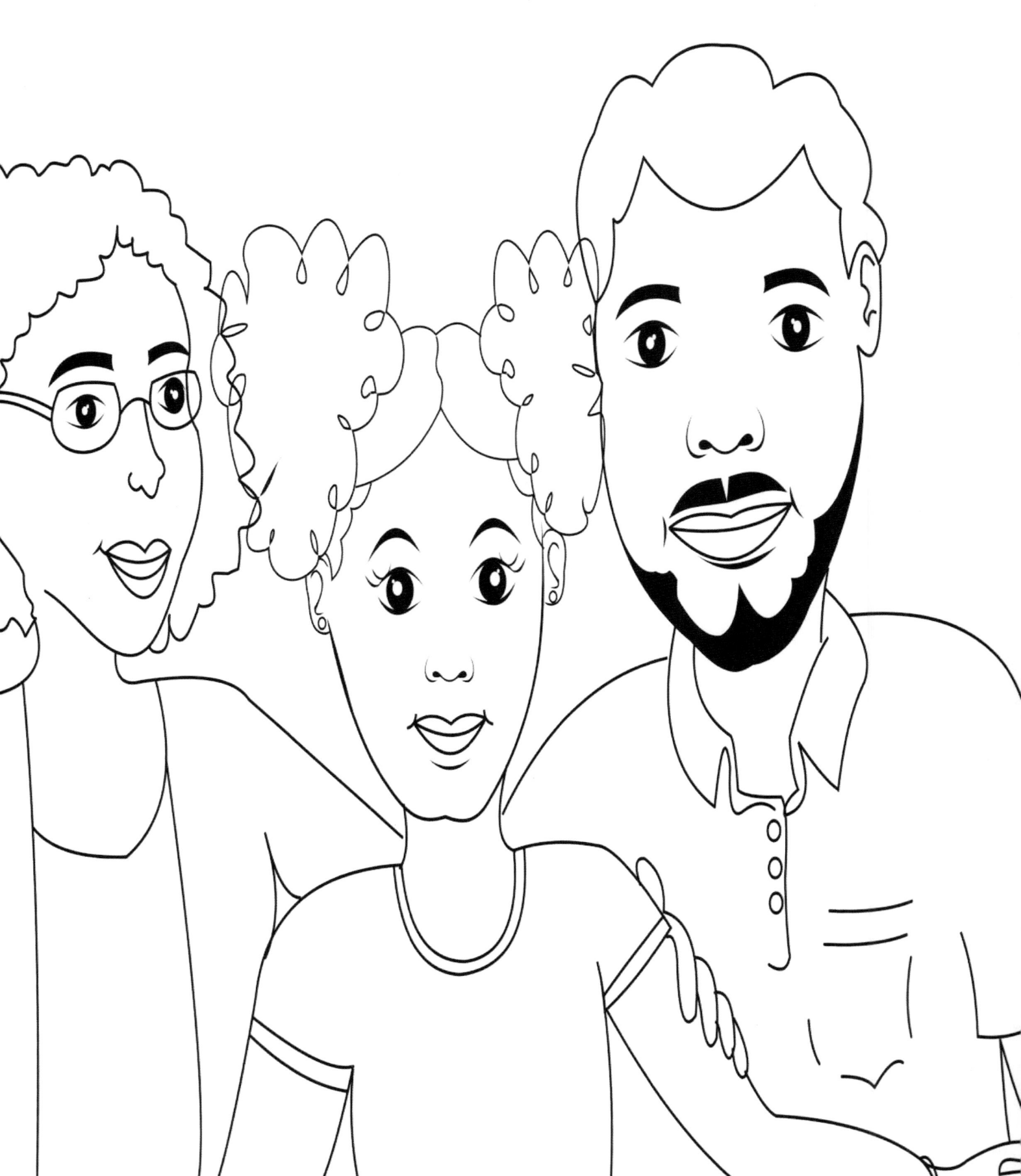

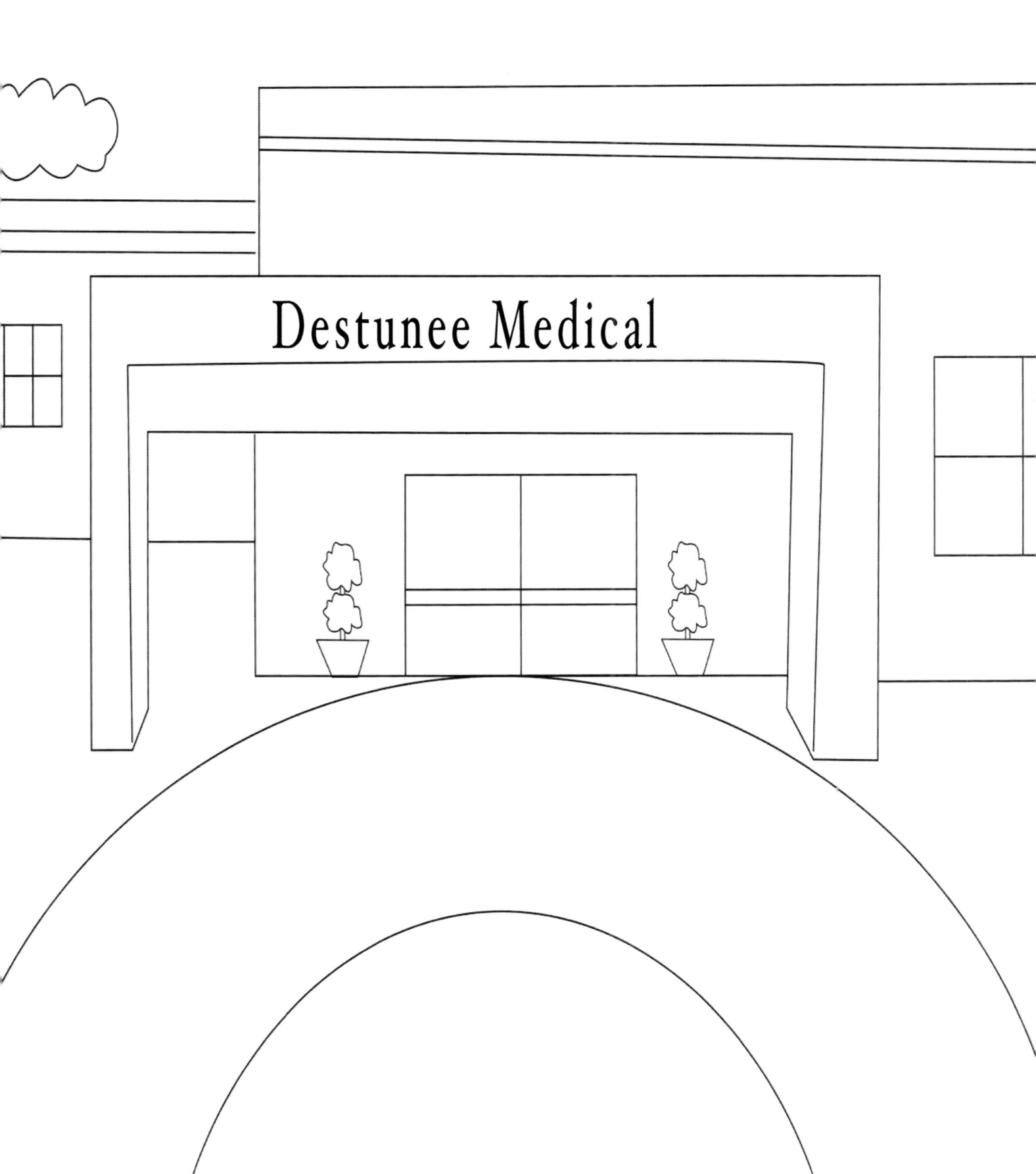

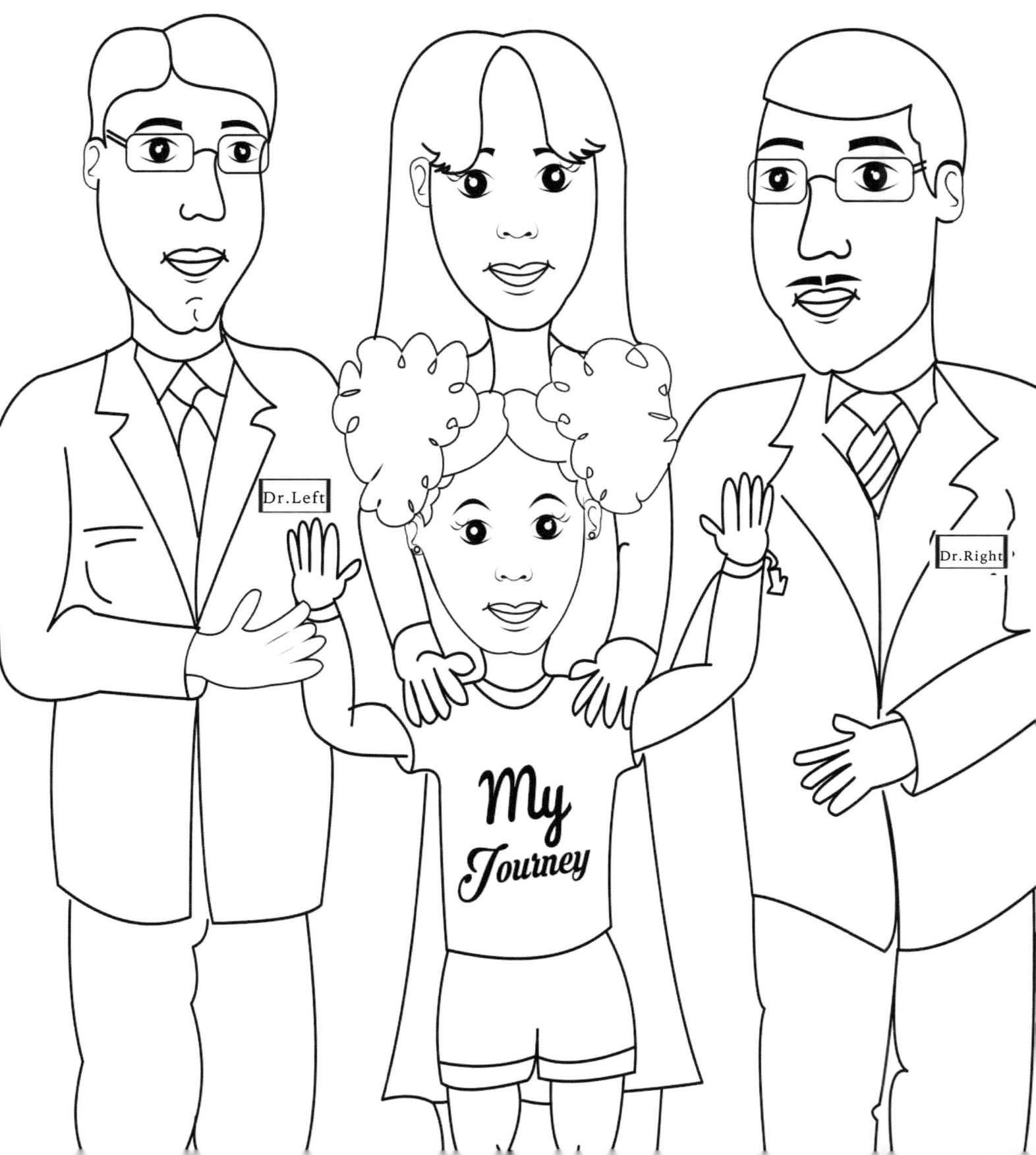

Printed in Great Britain
by Amazon